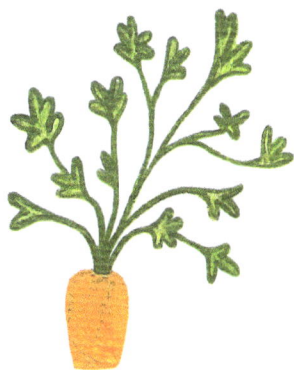 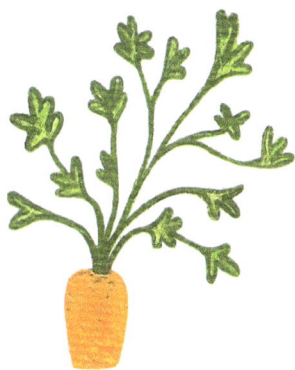 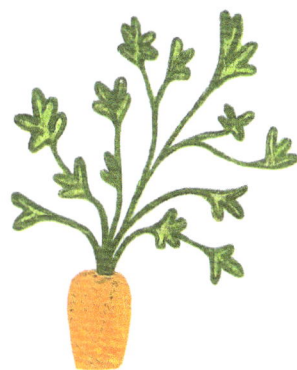

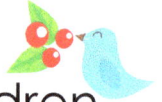

Wishing the best of health to our amazing children...
Kyle, Dylan, Jolena, Collin, Skylar, and Brynn,
and to children everywhere!

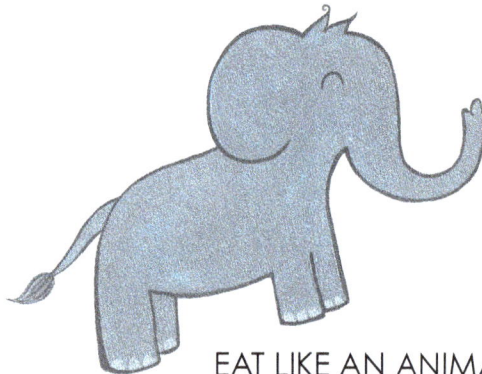

Published by Like An Animal Books, LLC, Branchburg, NJ 08876.
Library of Congress Control Number: 2017909416
ISBN-13: 978-0-692-90551-7
ISBN-10: 0-692-90551-0
Printed in the United States of America

$12.99

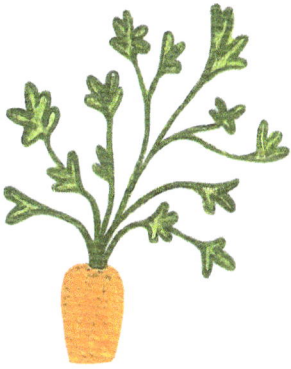

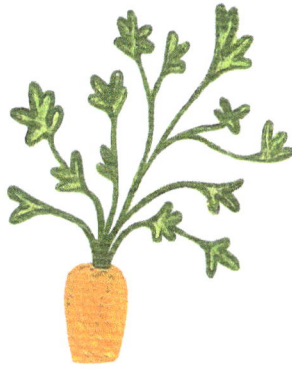

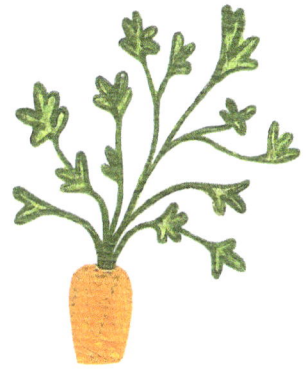

Fruits, vegetables, nuts, and seeds...
that's the way an animal feeds!

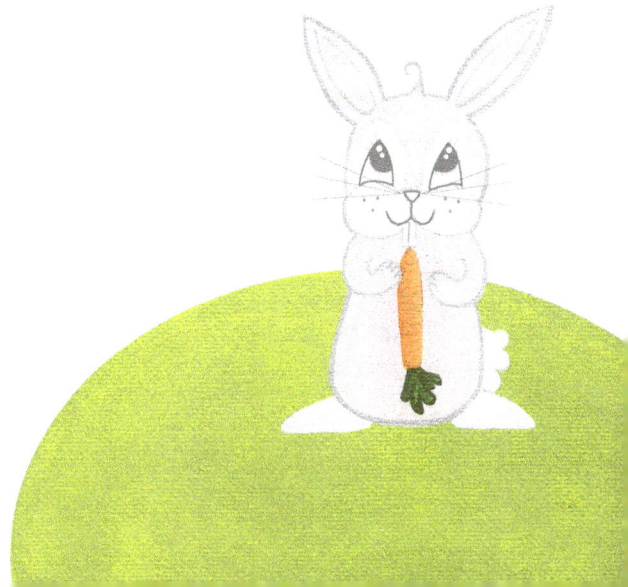

Monkey see,
monkey do...

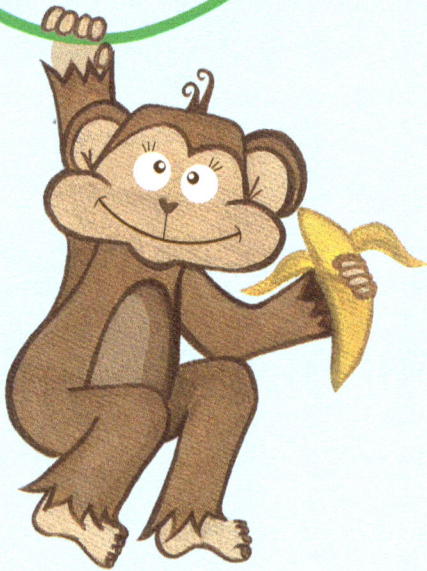

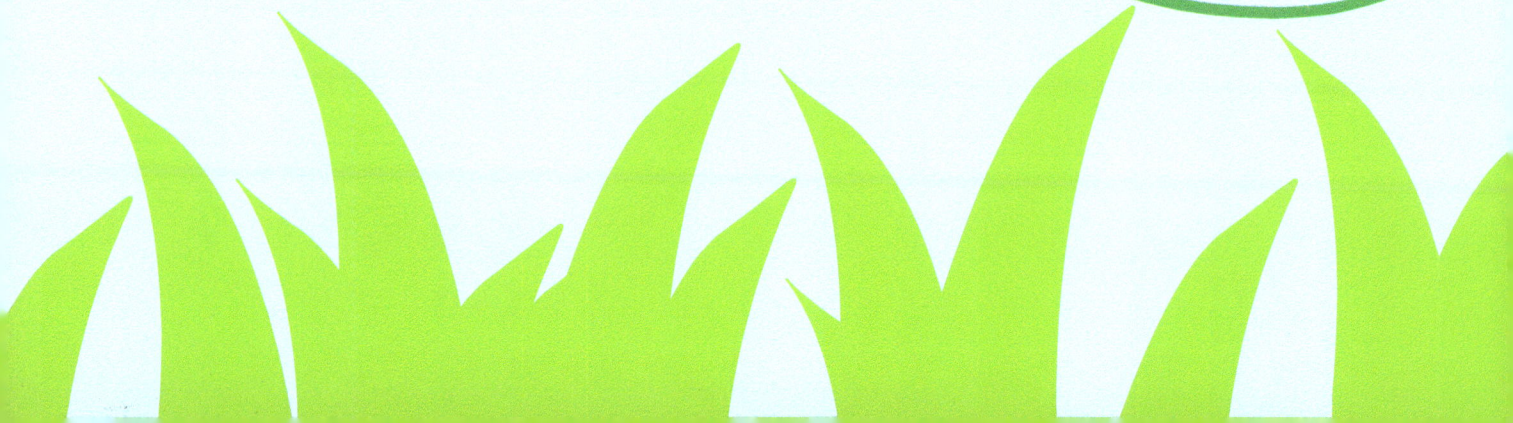

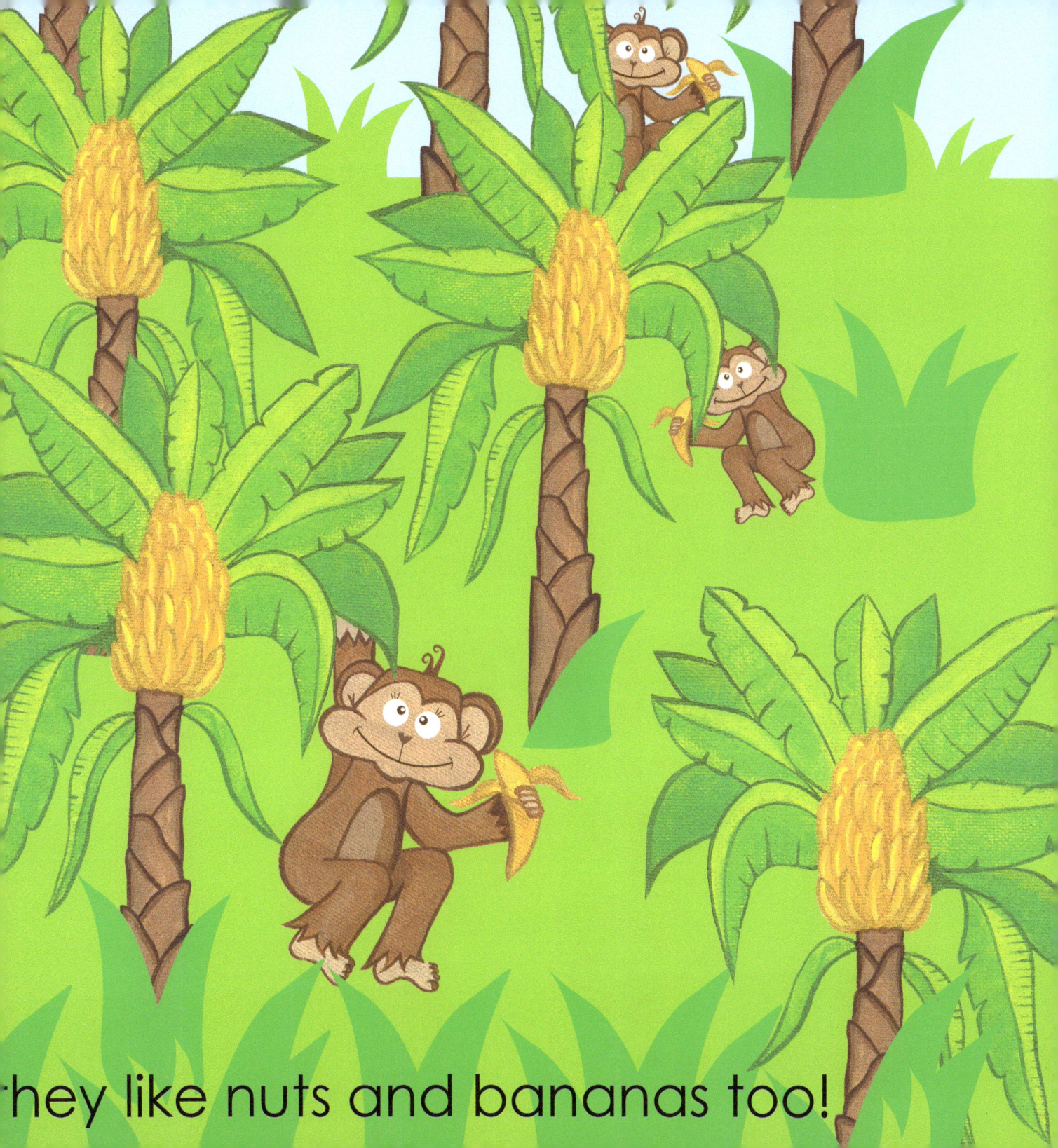

hey like nuts and bananas too!

A horse knows of course
about an apple a day...

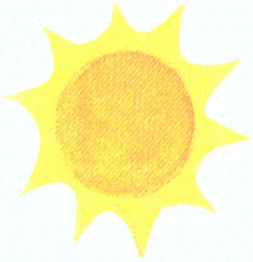

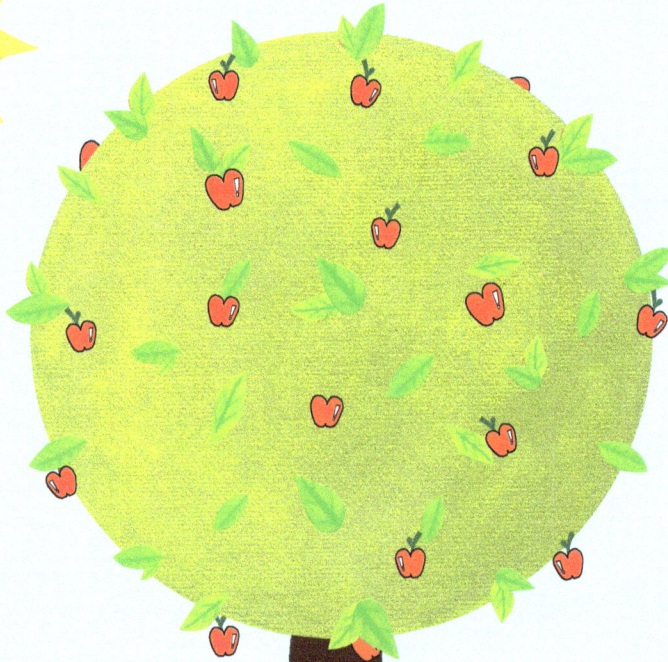

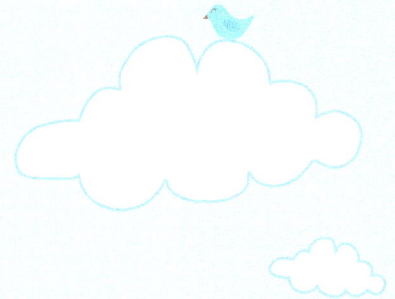

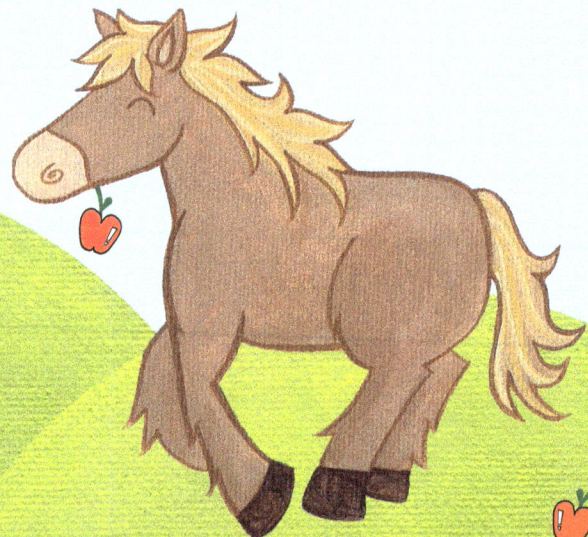

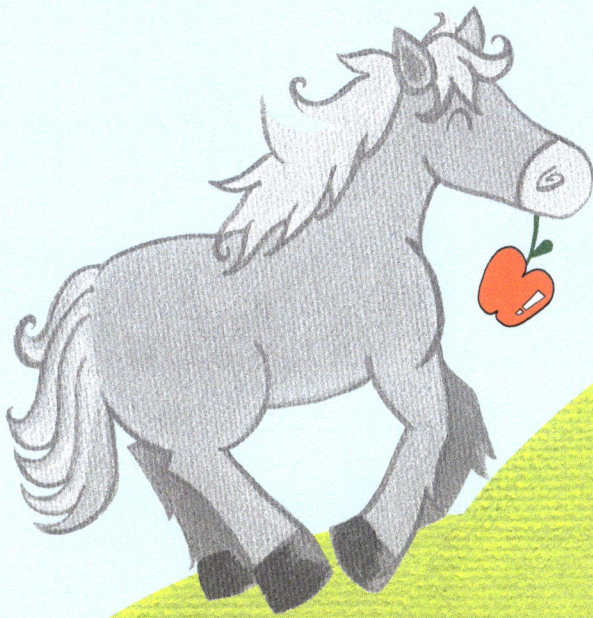

Neigh!

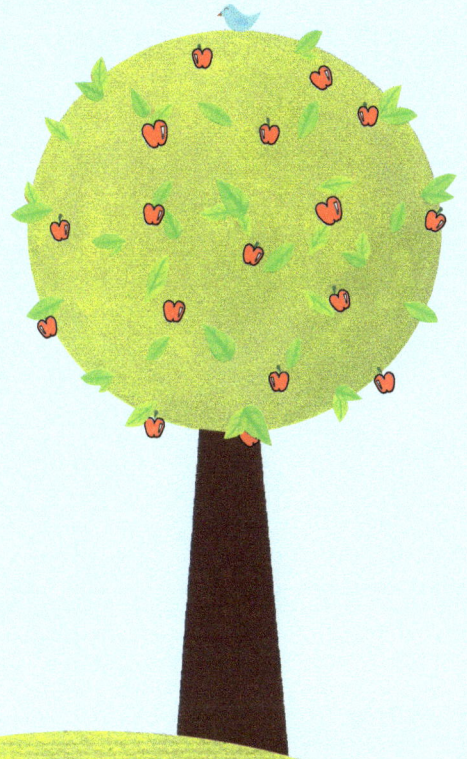

but if you ask him about it
he'll just neigh!

Birds eat seeds
and cherries too...

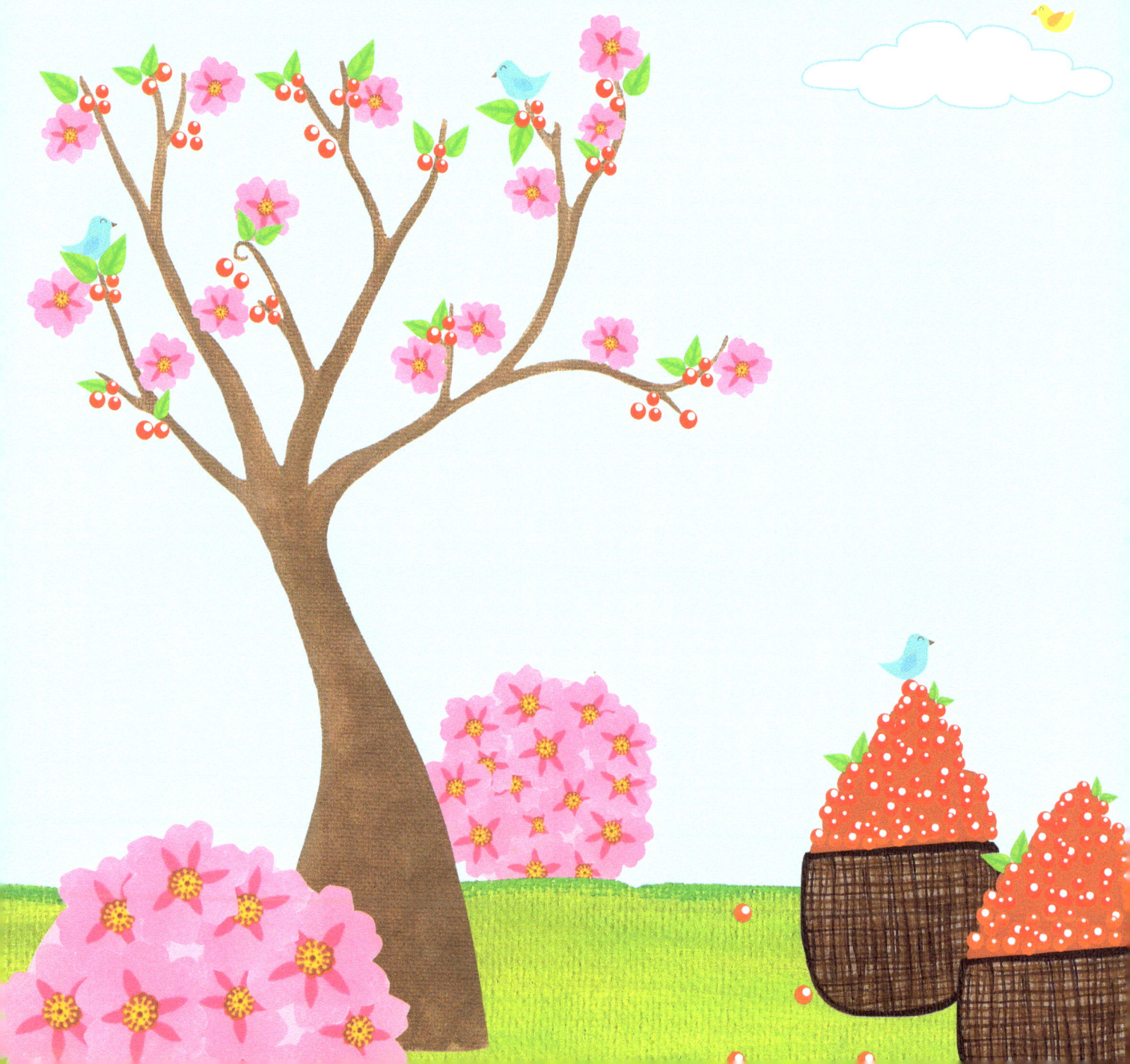

some might even say cuckoo!

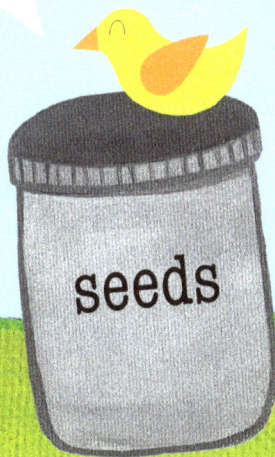

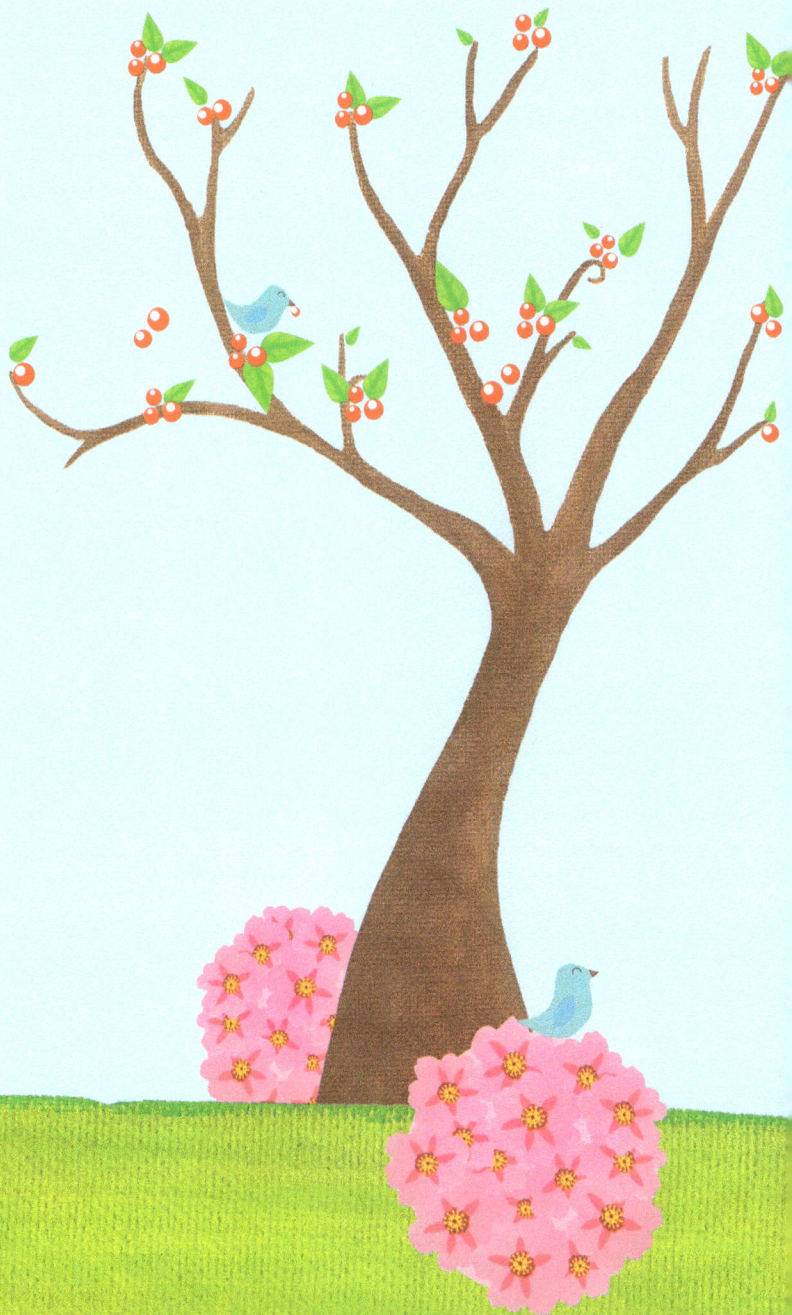

Rabbits like carrots, broccoli, and beans...

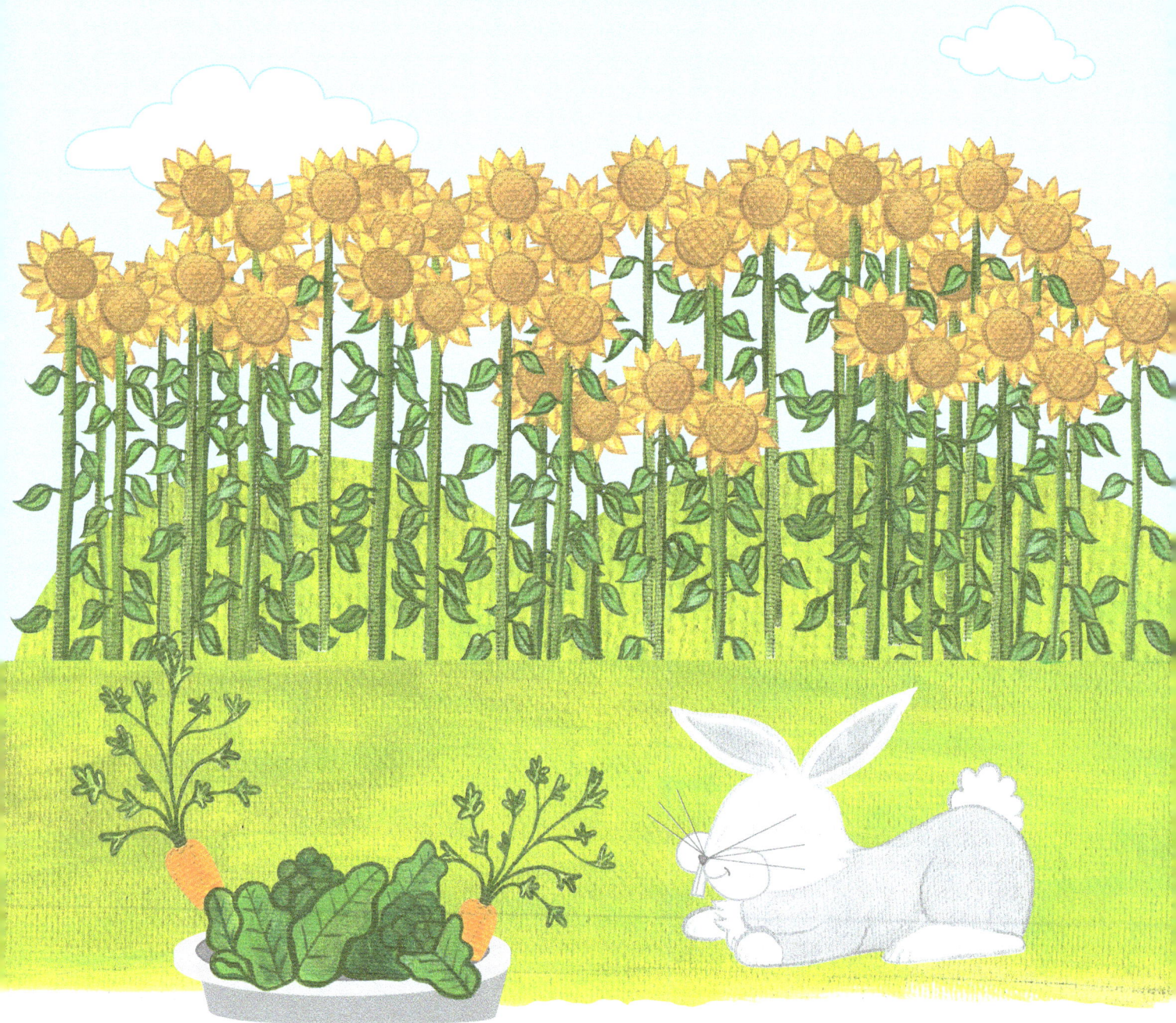

everything in our garden...
or so it seems!

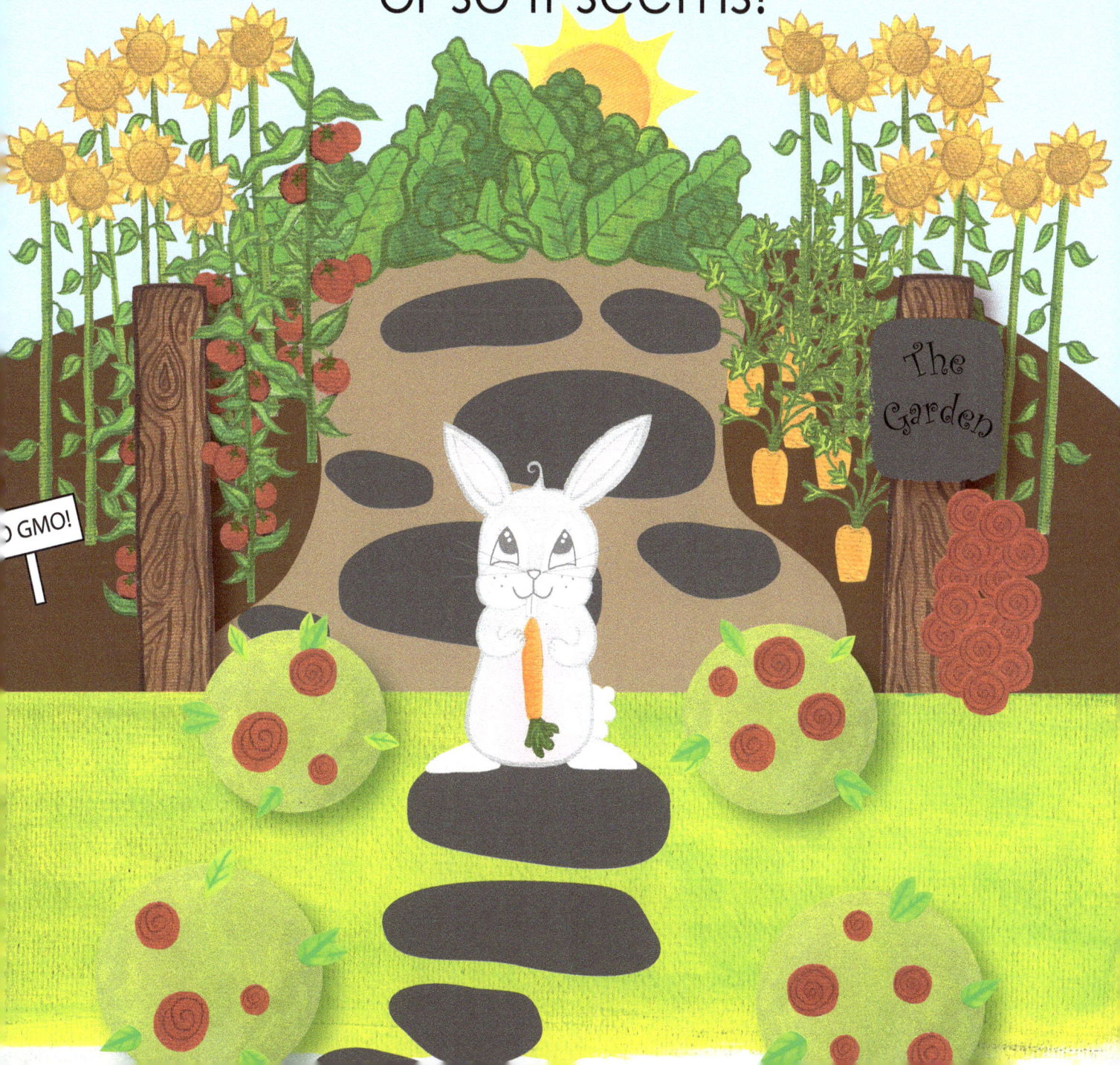

The Garden

GMO!

Elephants can eat an orange
in a single bite...

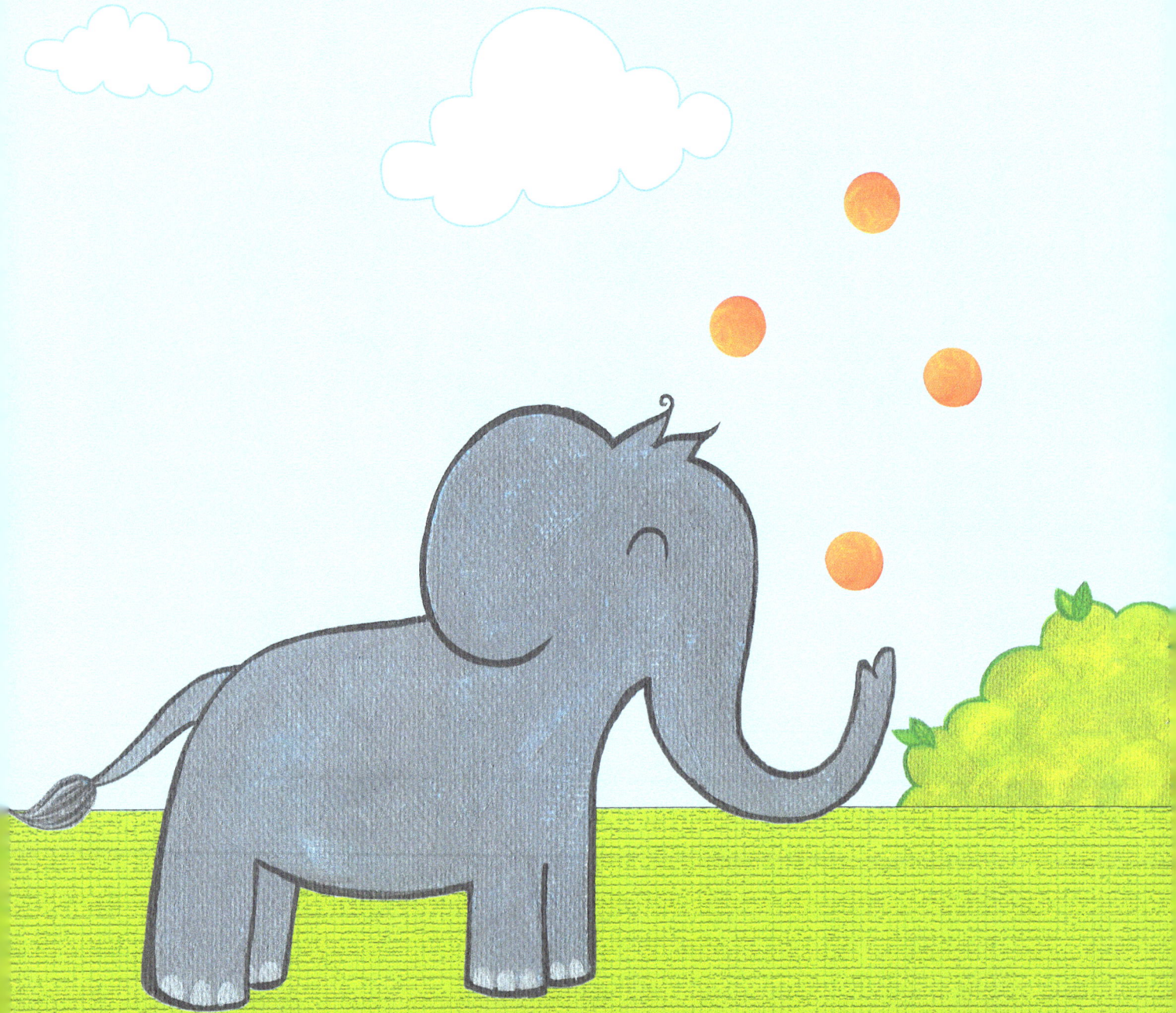

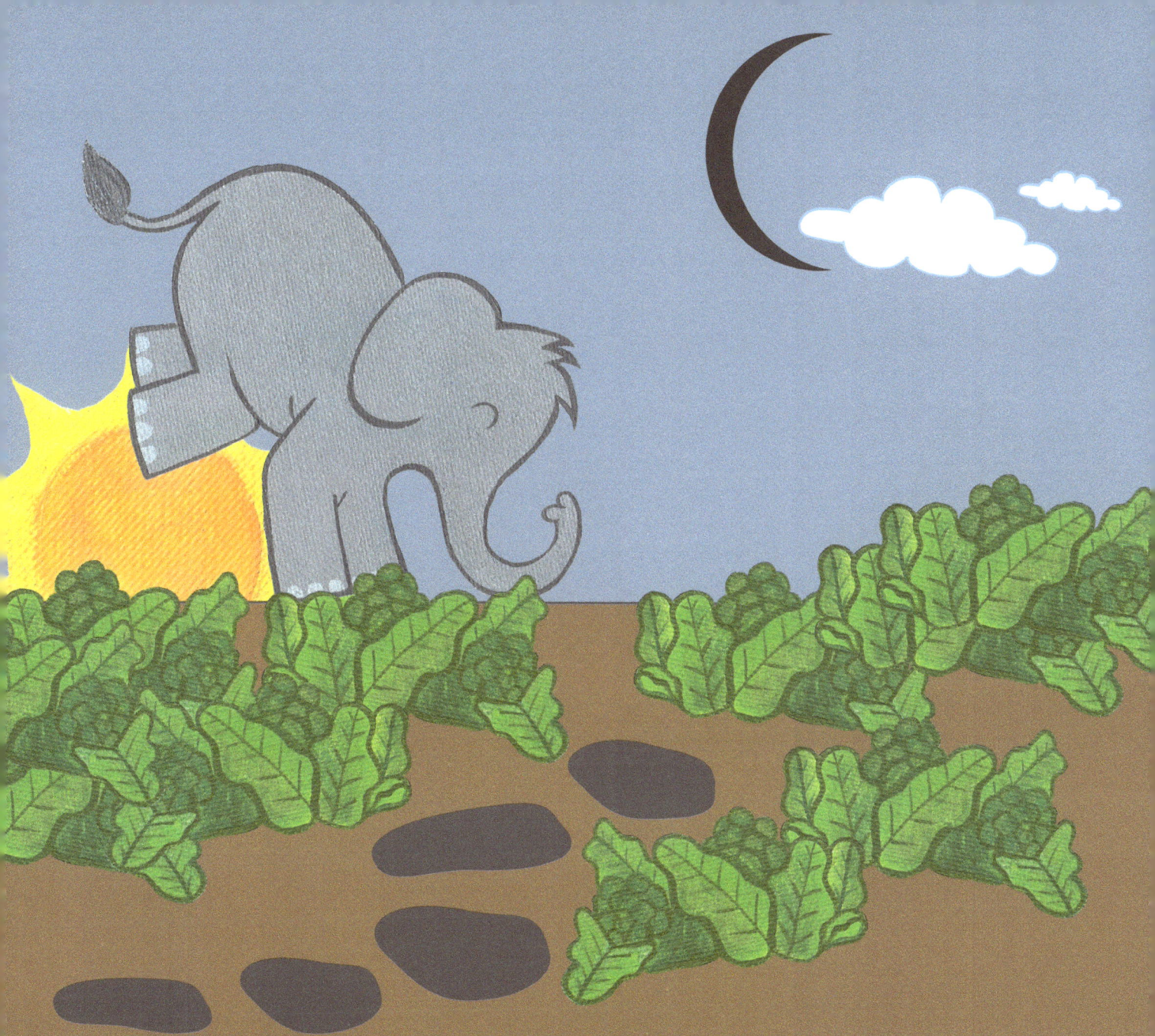

and munch on greens from
morning 'til night!

Bears picking blueberries
may seem funny...

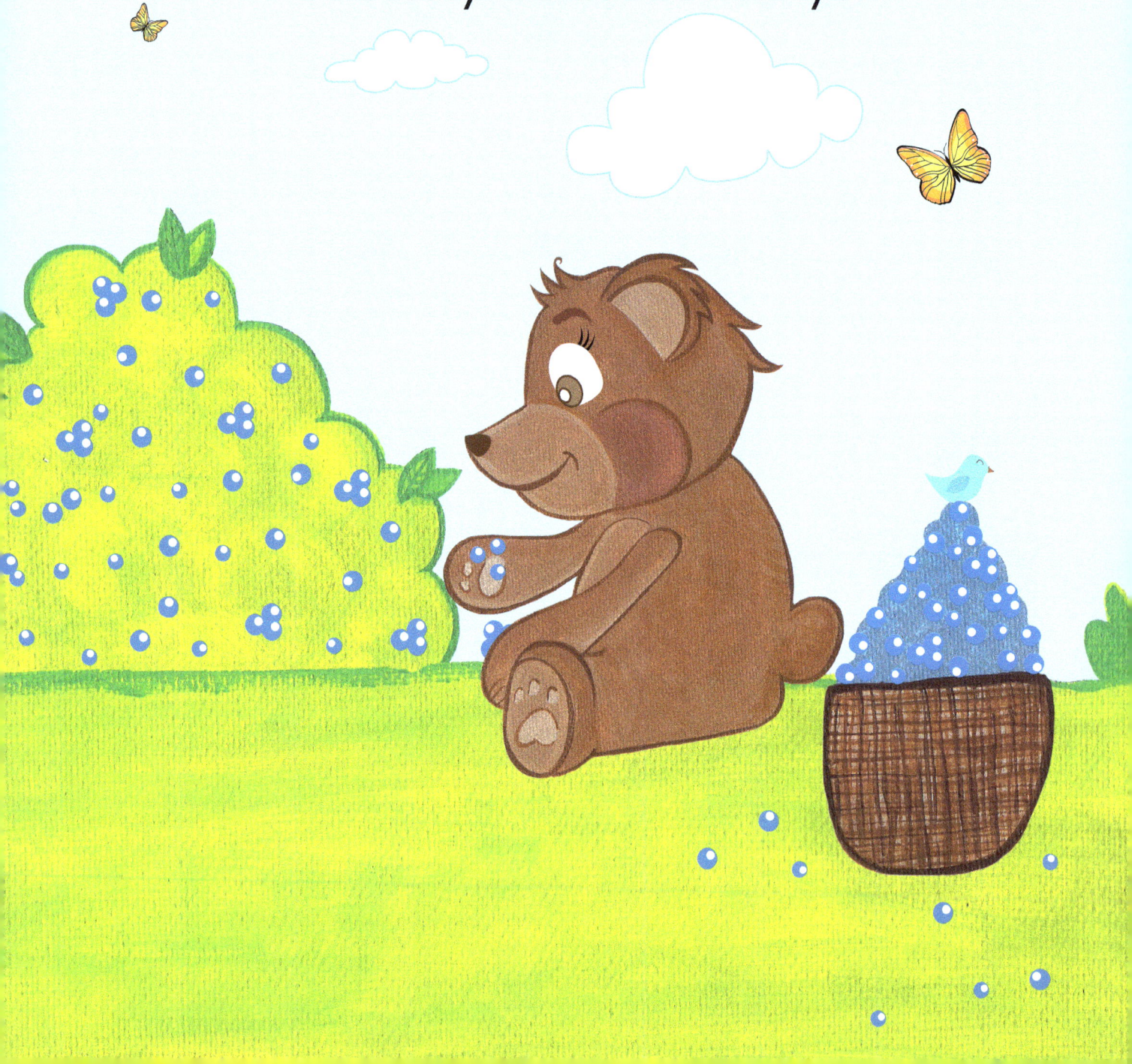

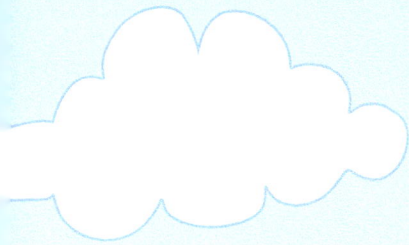

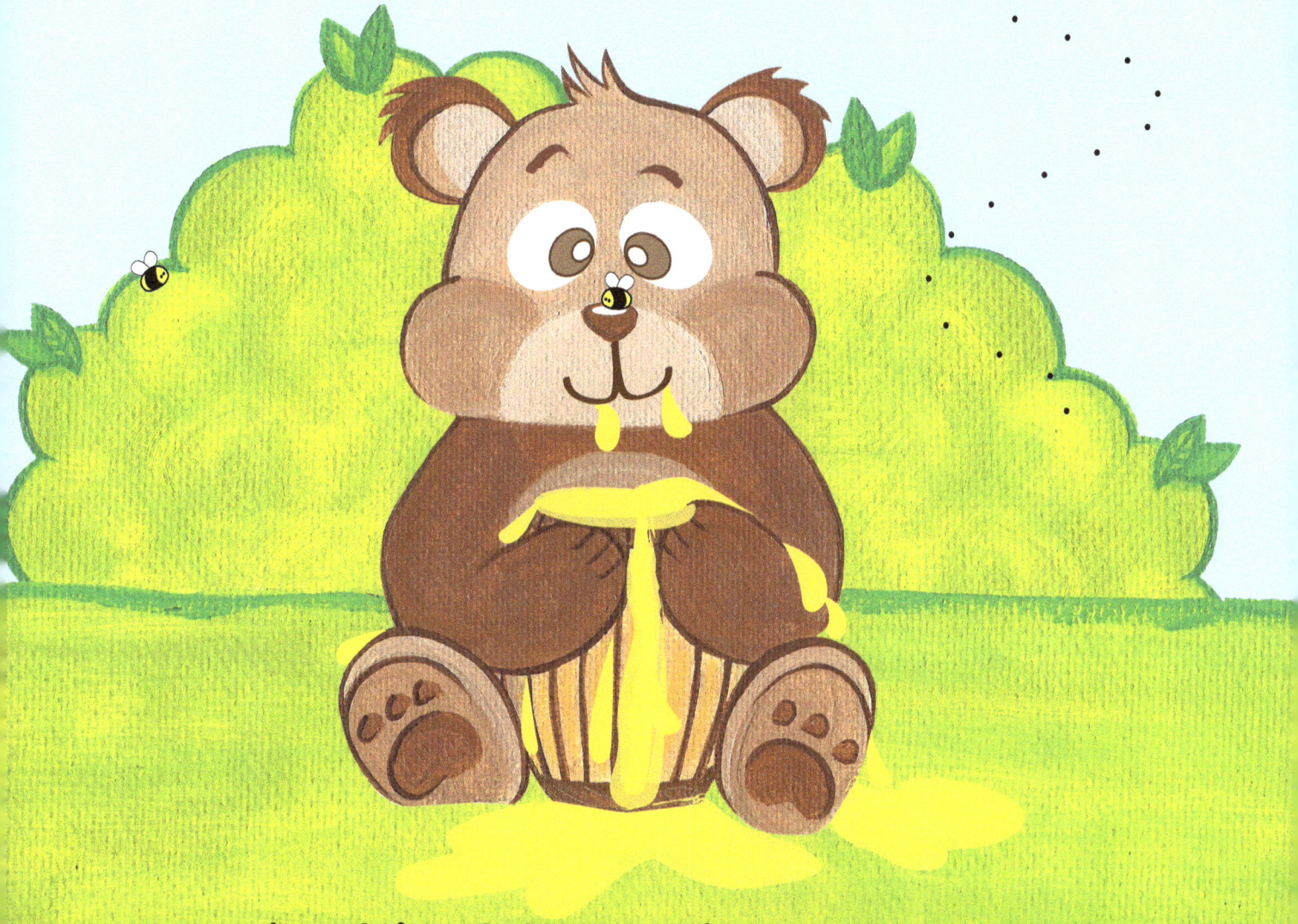

but just try to imagine
them sneaking some honey!

Some pigs are pink with curly tails...

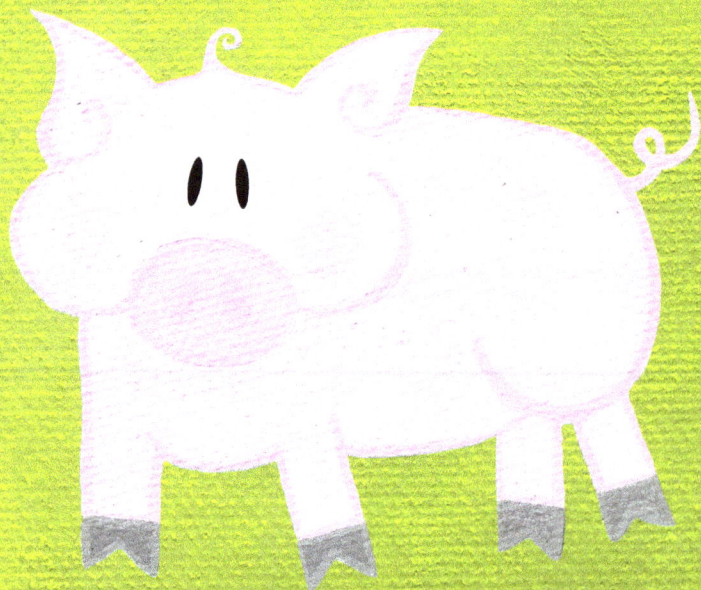

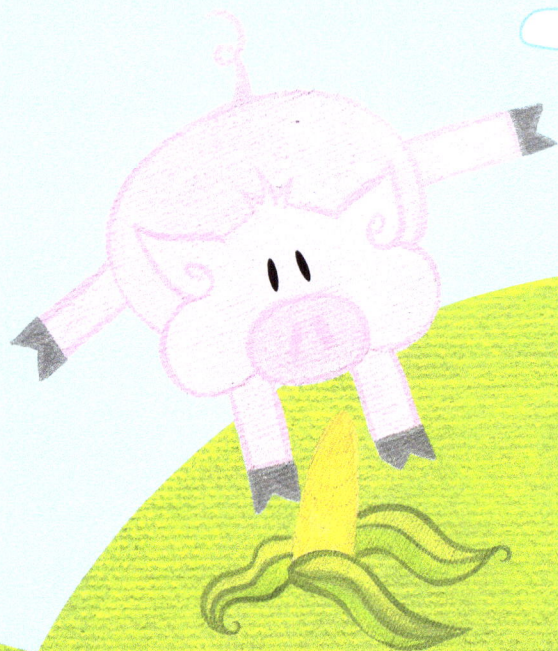

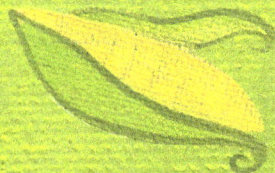

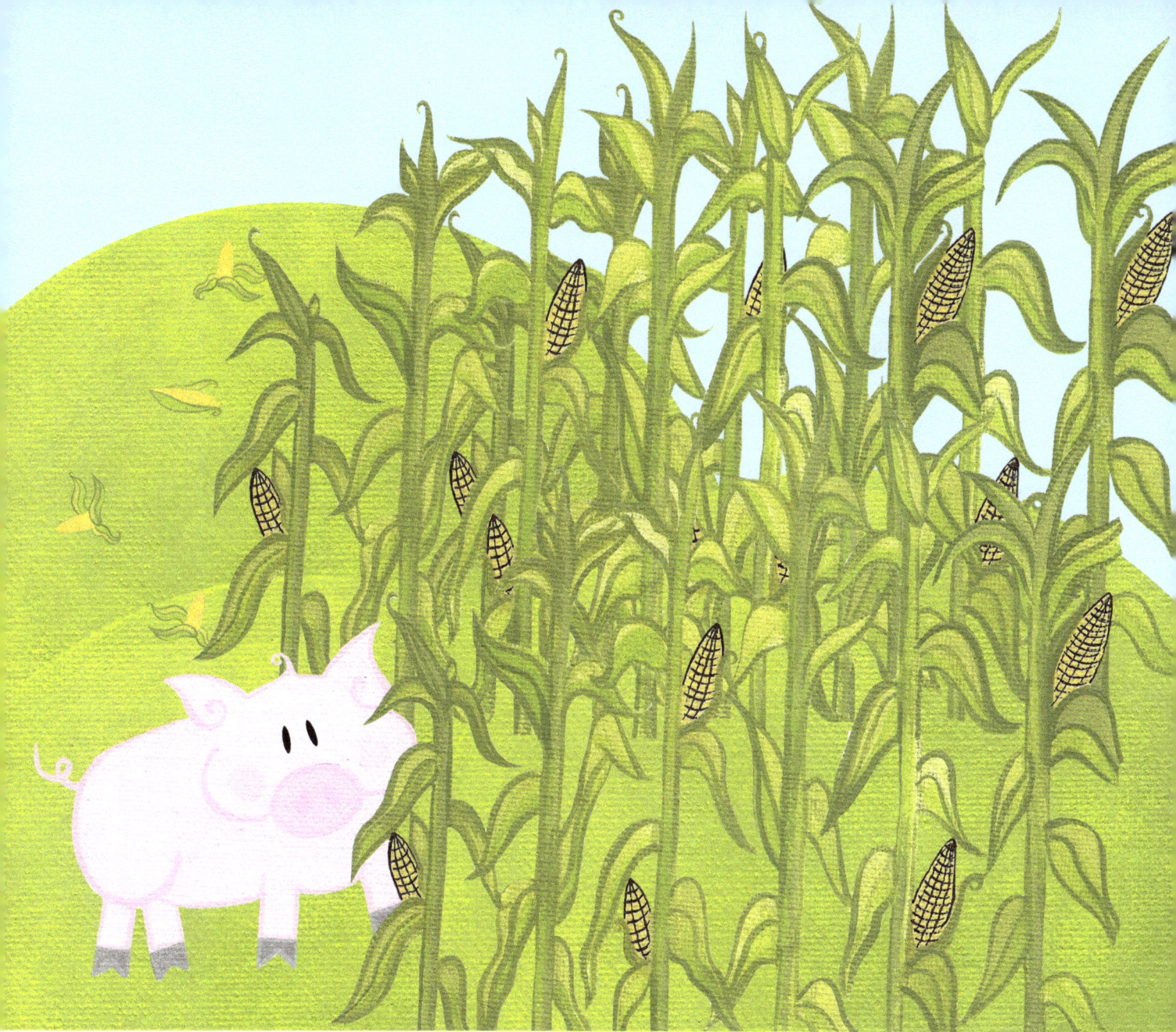

cobs of corn are in their trails!

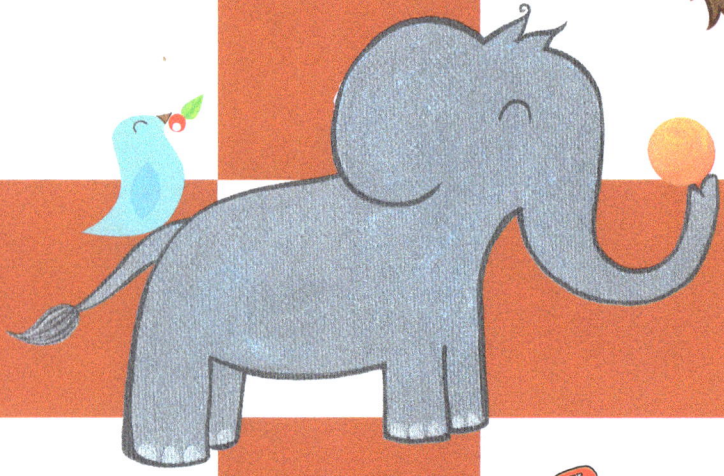

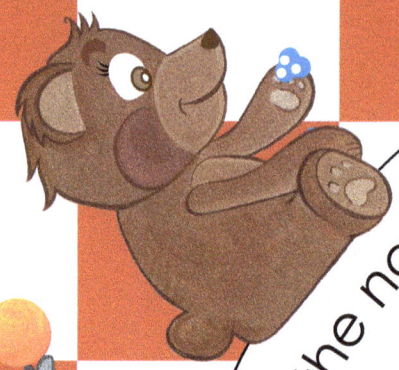

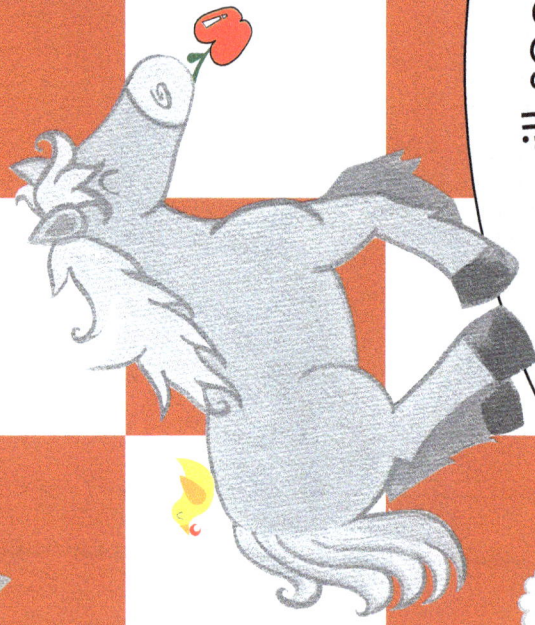

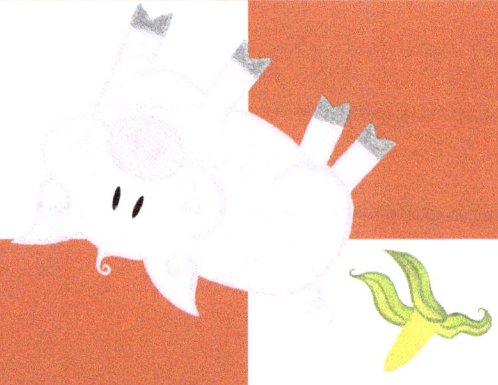

Eat like an animal and you will see, that it's the natural way to be!

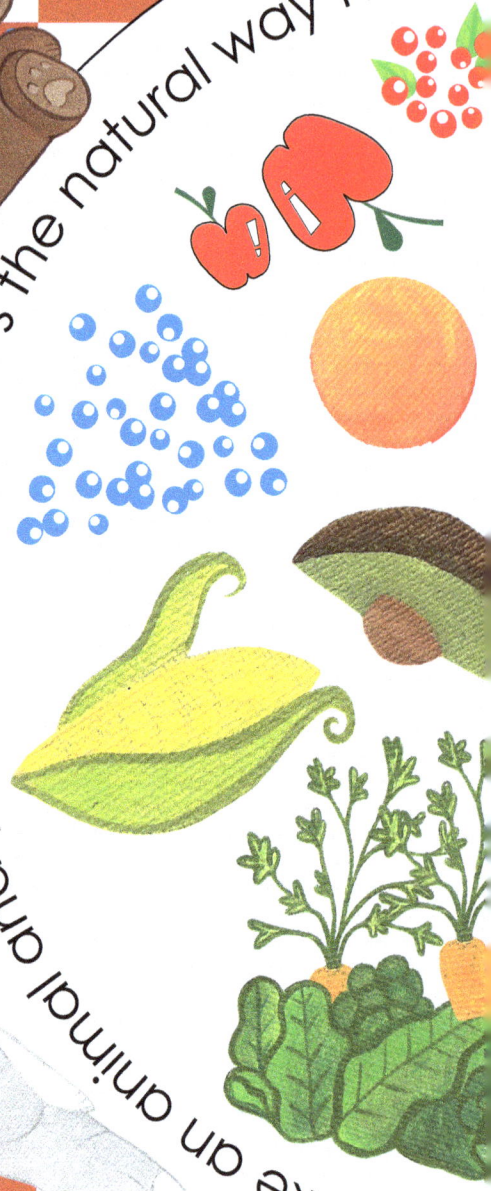

Now that you know what animals do, you can act like an animal too

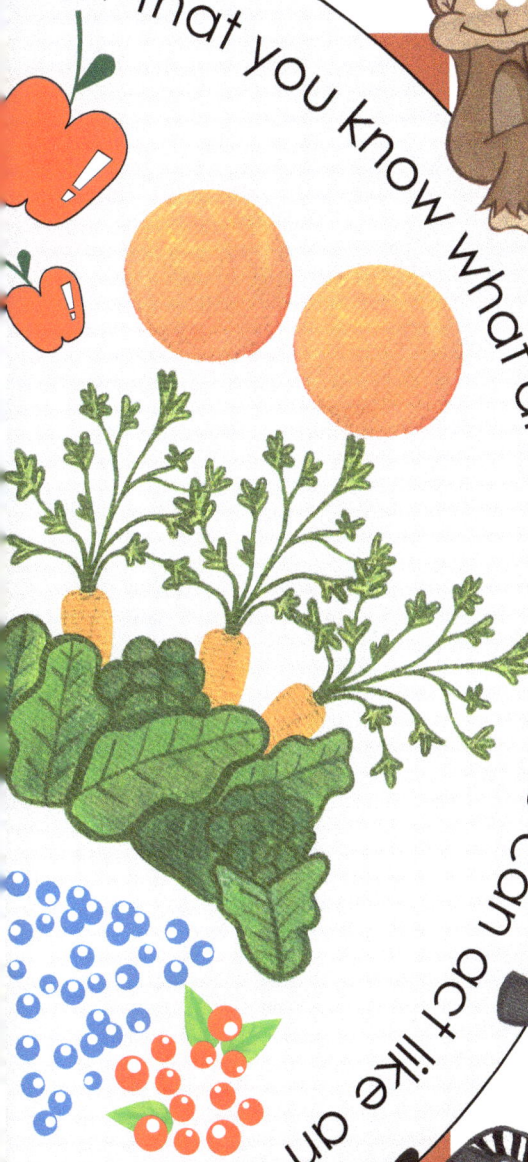

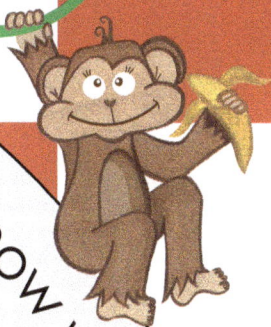

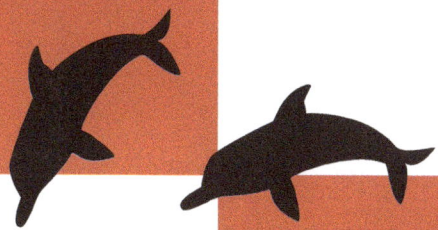

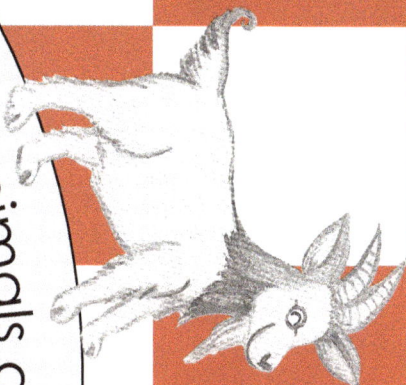

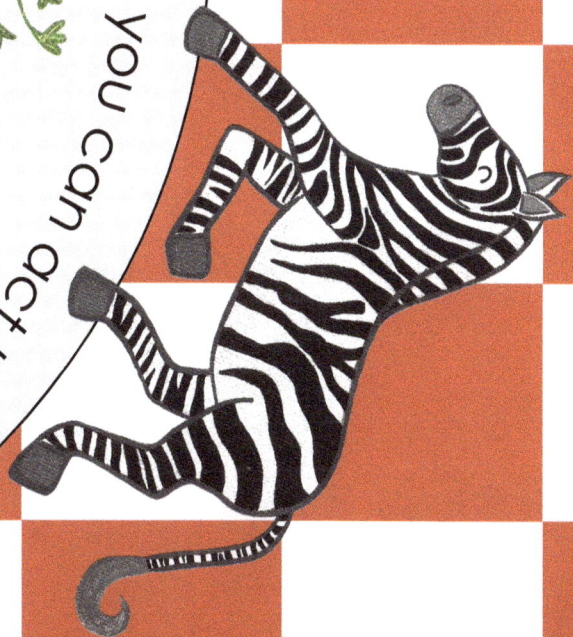

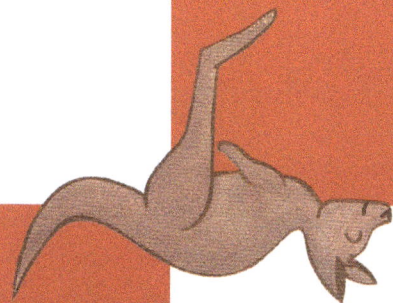

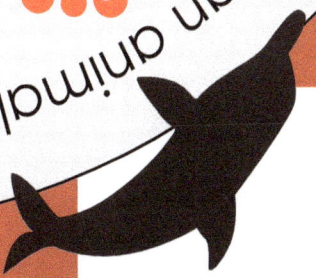

jumping and chasing the sun
from the day!

During sunset dolphins play...

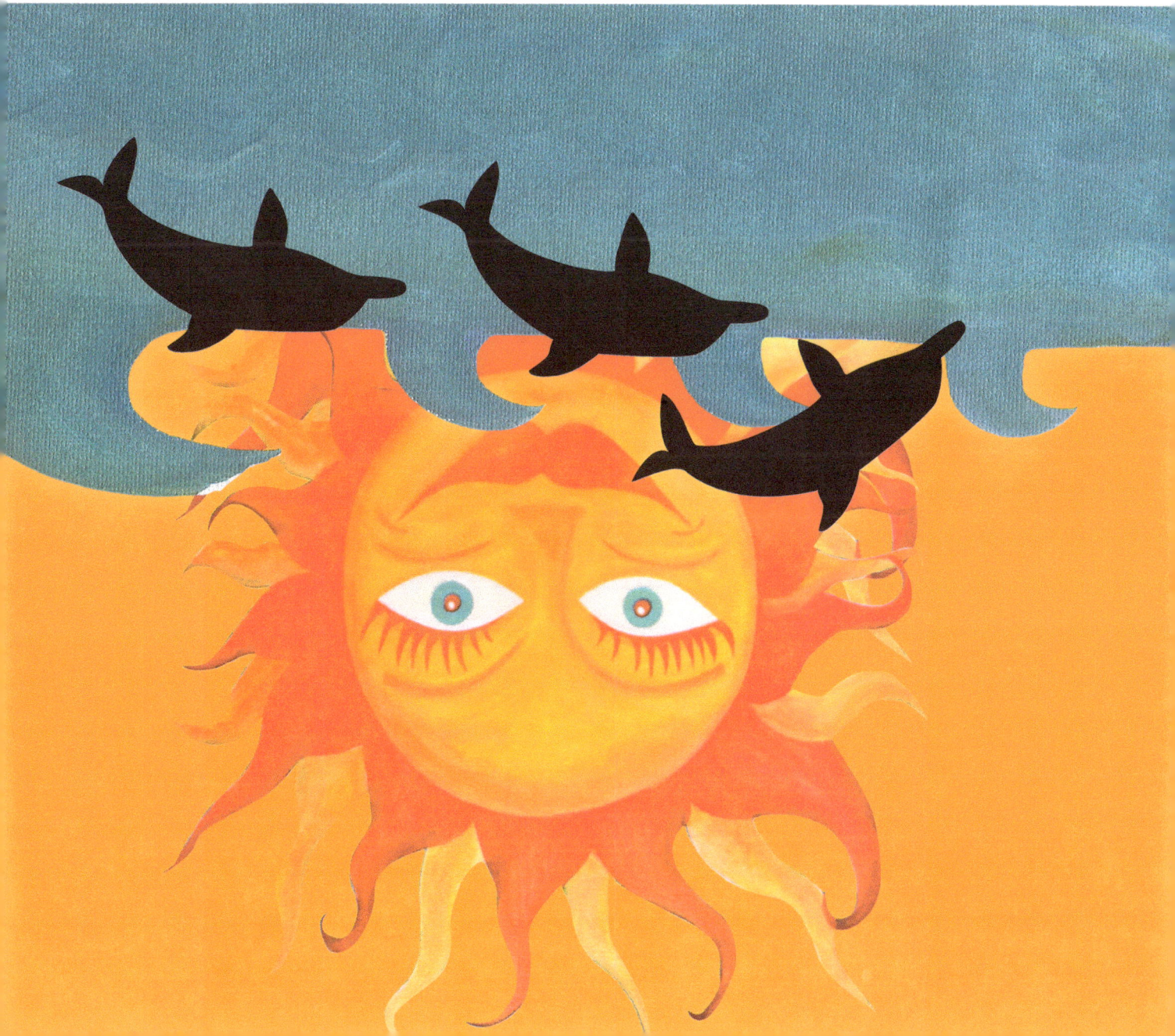

loving to run whether it's cold or hot!

A horse will gallop, walk, and trot...

to get to the top,
or just for the thrill!

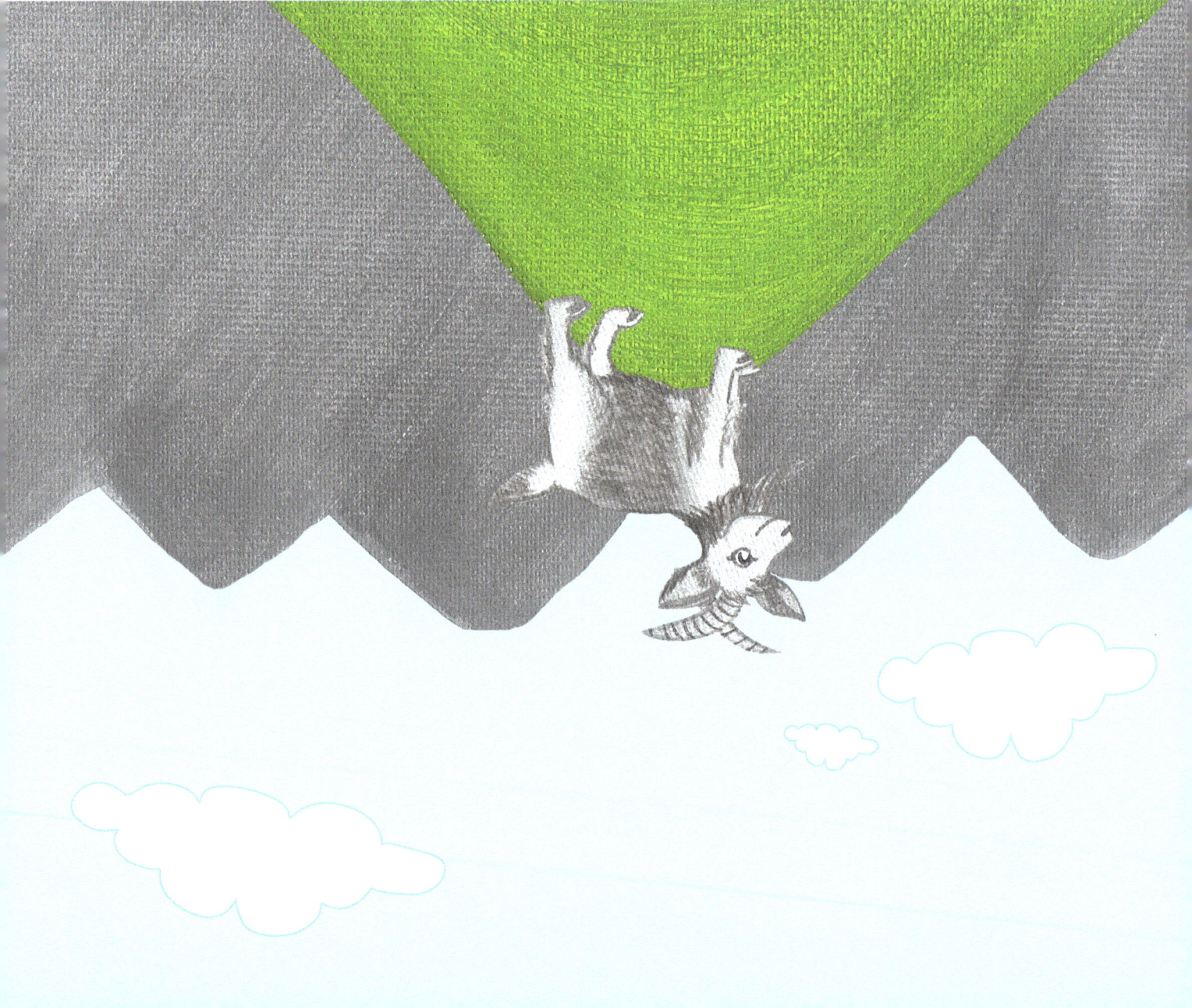

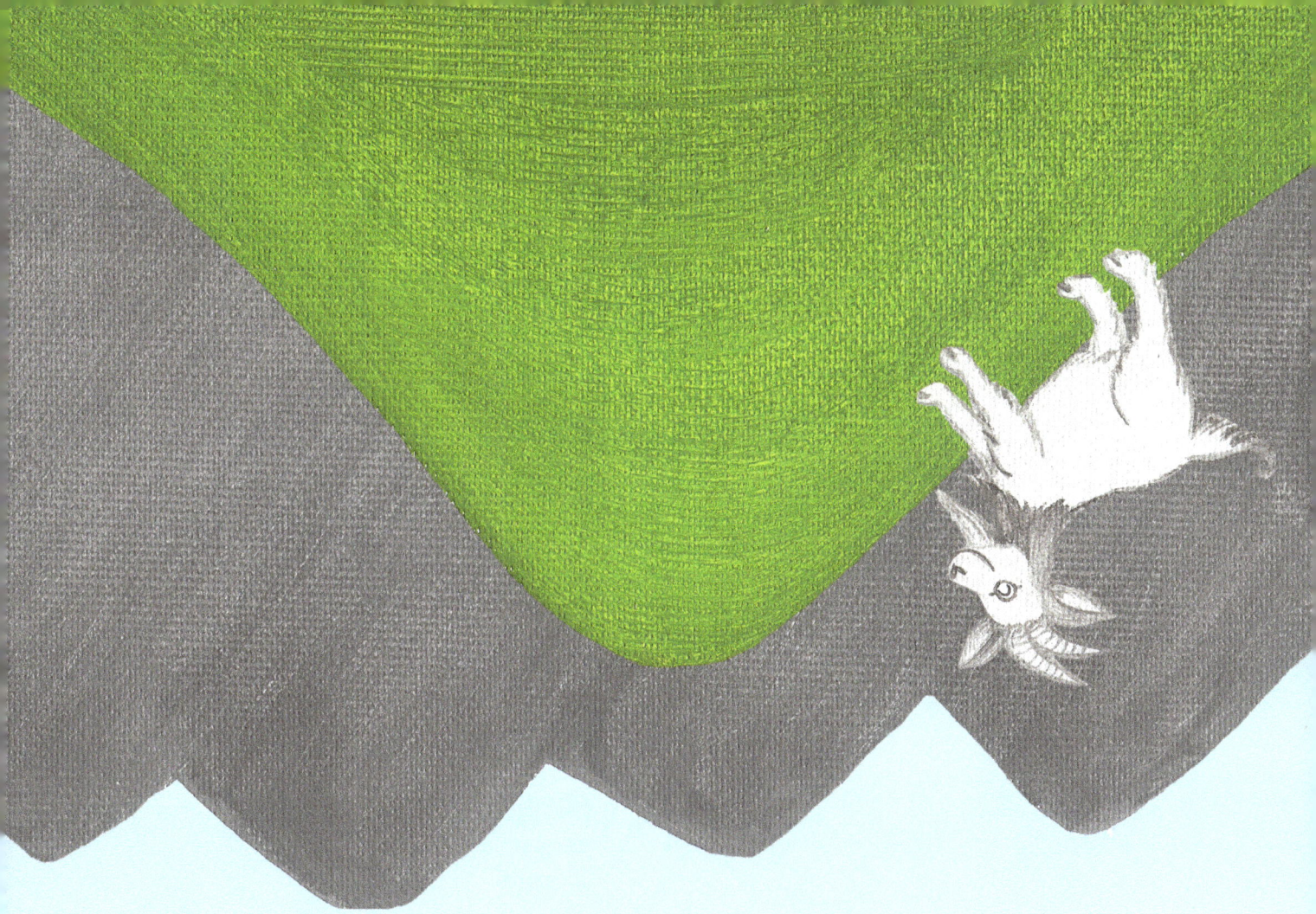

A goat has a beard and
can climb a steep hill...

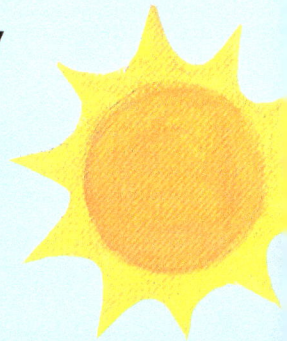

here's nothing like a fast-paced chase!

Across the fields zebras leap and race.

and never, ever seems to stop!

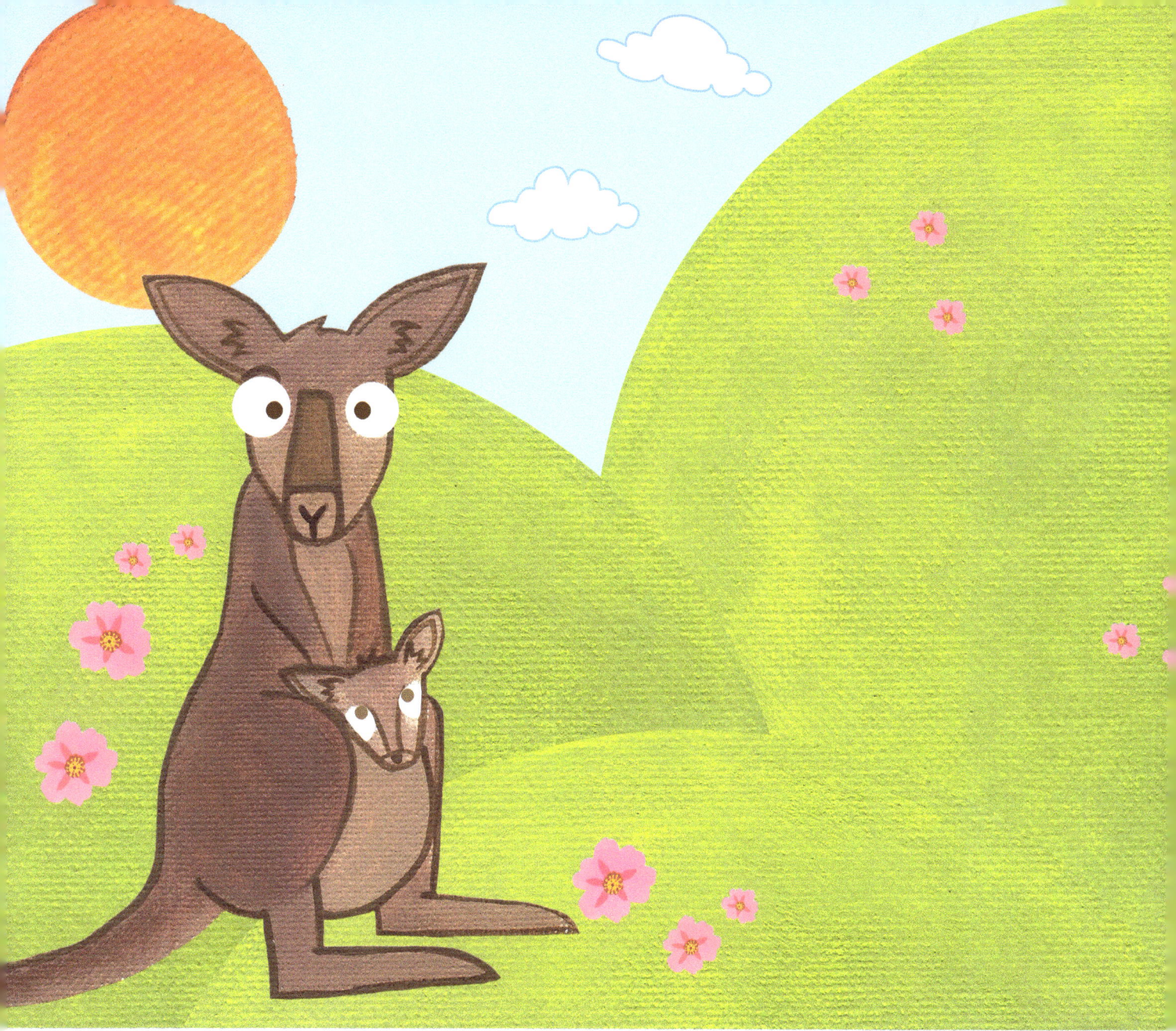

A kangaroo likes to hop and hop...

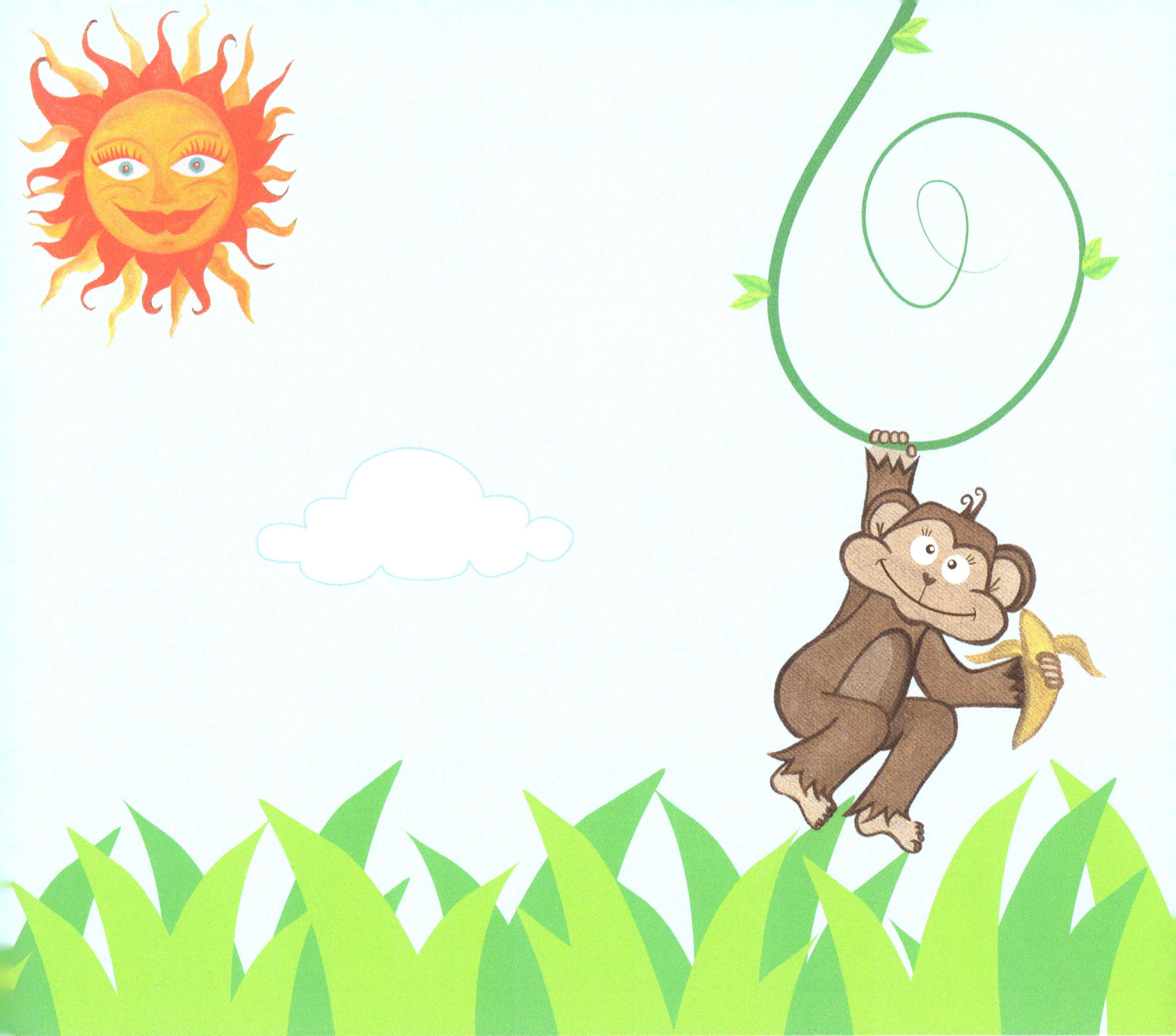

a monkey swinging happily!

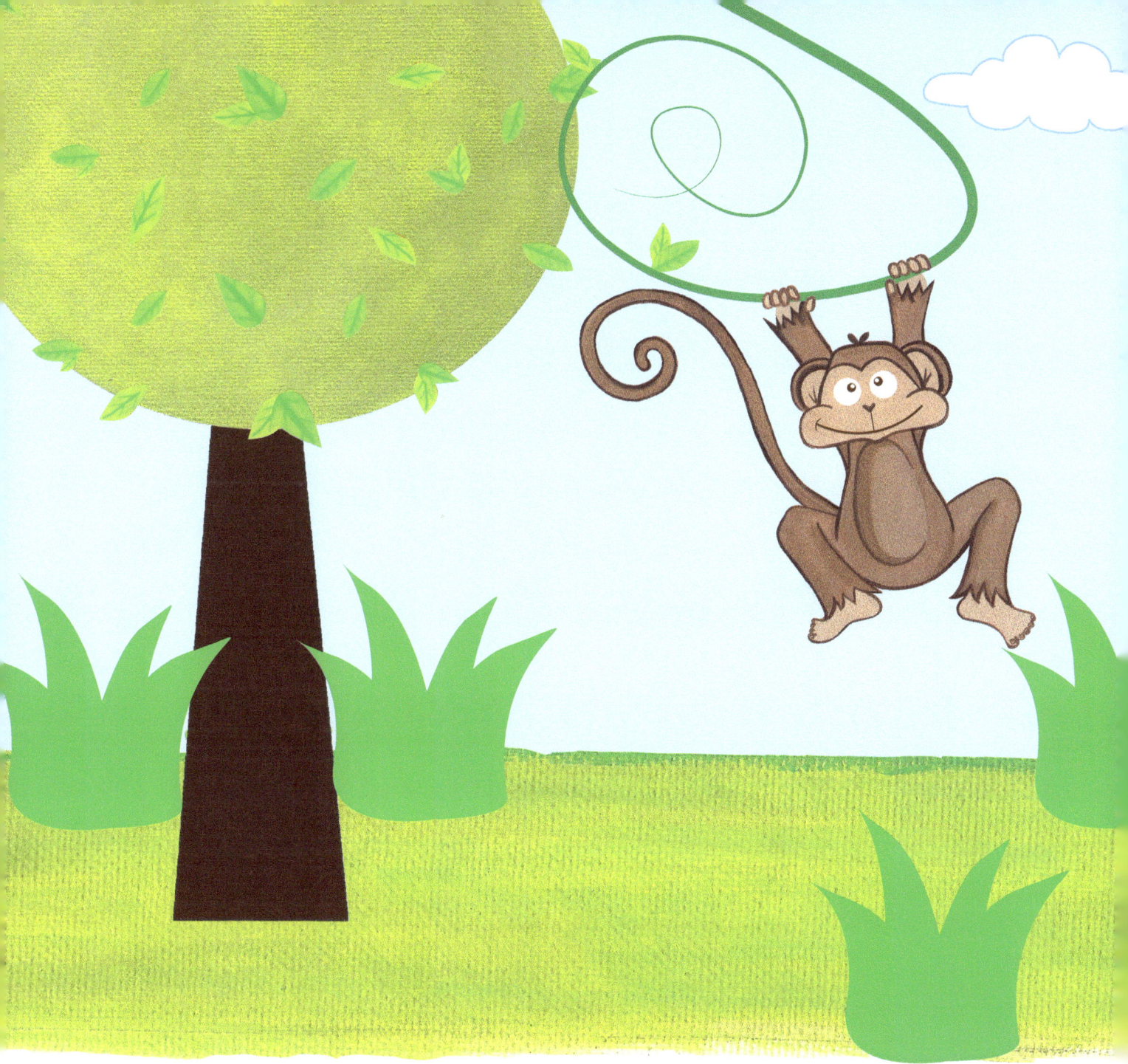

From tree to tree, you can see...

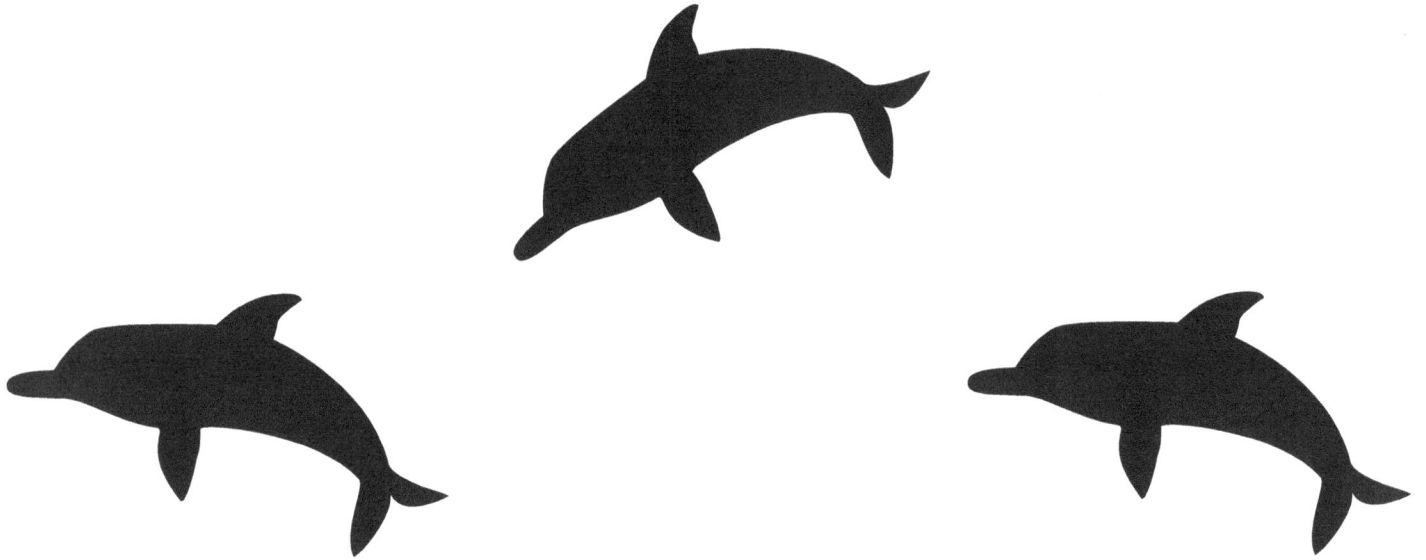

Jump, swim, hop, and run...
that's the way an animal has fun!

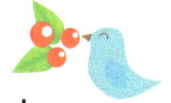

Wishing the best of health to our amazing children...
Kyle, Dylan, Jolena, Collin, Skylar, and Brynn,
and to children everywhere!

As running partners and medical writers, Linda J. Lipp and Dawn Hartman Chiu co-wrote the **Eat Like an Animal** and **Act Like an Animal** books to inspire others to make positive lifestyle changes and to help prevent obesity and type 2 diabetes in children. Rachel Lee Cronin, an artist, yoga instructor, and health enthusiast brought this vision to life by creating colorful and engaging illustrations. As moms, they hope their efforts will inspire children to mimic the behaviors of the animals featured in the books by eating healthful foods and being active on a regular basis!

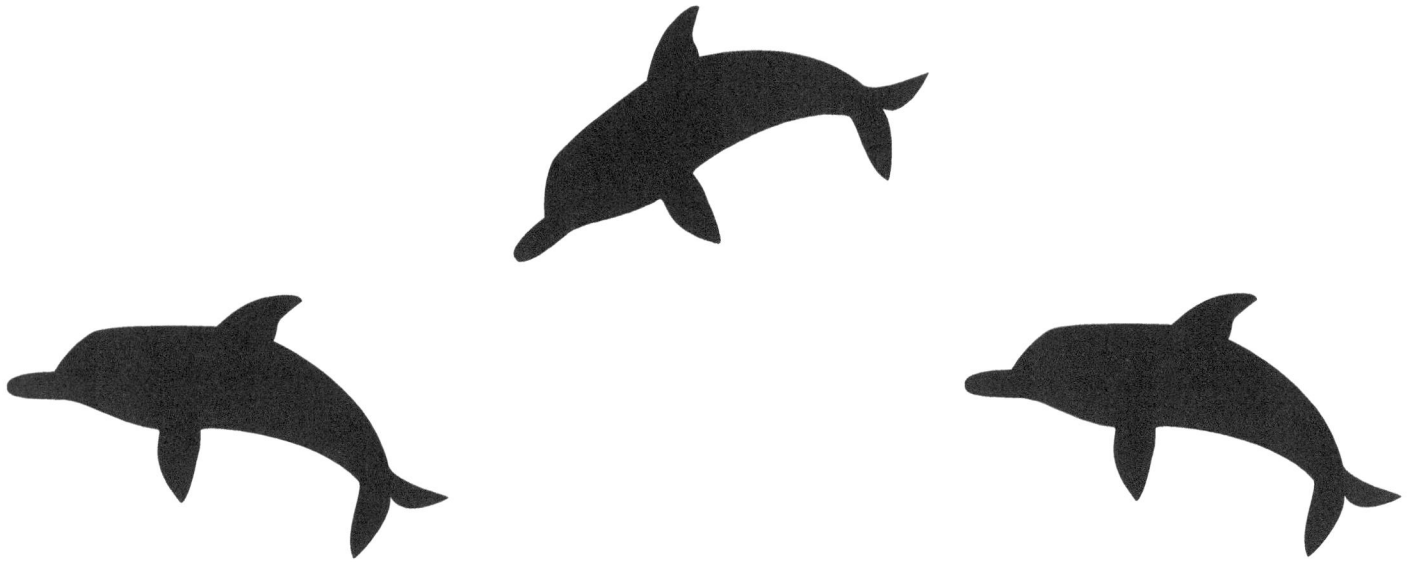

www.ingramcontent.com/pod-product-compliance
Lightning Source LLC
Chambersburg PA
CBHW051612030426

42334CB00035B/3496